Homemade Cleaners

50 DIY Cleaners Recipes for Your Home

Introduction

DIY cleaning products are good and improve your health. These cleaning products will keep your environment clean because these are free from toxins. If you have children in your house, commercial cleaning products can be really dangerous for you.

It is important to keep them away from your children, but it is difficult to keep commercial cleaners away from children. Kids are really curious about everything and you can get the advantage of organic cleaning products. These healthy products are better for everyone because of zero toxins. If you have children in your house, you should have them. It will be good to make one cabinet in your house and put all cleaning products in this cabinet.

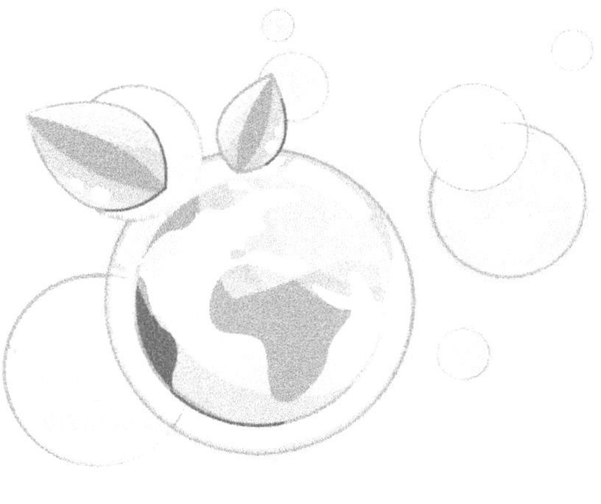

These products are good to improve your health and you can protect your environment too with the help of these products. If you want these green cleaners, you can follow the 50 recipes given in this book. These recipes have natural ingredients and these are perfectly safe for each and every person.

You can use a few basic ingredients available at your home to make these chemicals. These are good for your house and family members. These recipes will help you to prepare your own cleaners and get rid of chemicals full of chemicals. There are 50 recipes to prepare your own products, such as cleaners, dishwasher, shampoo, detergents and soap.

Chapter 1 – DIY Cleaning Products for Home

You should keep your home clean without any product full of chemical. There are a few recipes for everyone:

Recipe 01: Liquid Personal Soap

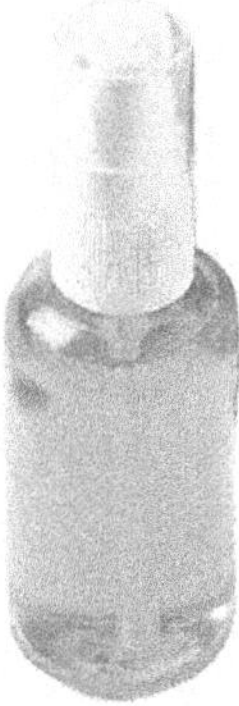

- 6 oz distilled water
- 7 oz coconut oil
- 16.5 oz olive oil
- 16.5 oz distilled or filtered water
- 5.5 oz potassium hydroxide
- 40 oz distilled water
- 3 oz borax
- Essential Oil (100 percent pure)
- Color

Directions:

Before starting work, you have to measure all ingredients carefully.

Measure the olive and coconut oil and keep them in the slow cooker. Set the cooker on the low setting. Take a quart jar and weight water in it. Slowly include an accurate quantity of potassium hydroxide and stir with a stick. There would be a sound for some reaction.

The potassium hydroxide solution will appear clear and you may add water mixture to the oils. There is no need to worry about the temperature. Carefully mix it for five minutes so that the oils and potassium may make a perfect blend. After five minutes, use a stick blender to mix and wait for 30 minutes to get a trace. At the trace stage, the mixture will be thick like pudding.

Cook it in the slow cooker for 30 minutes with a lid on and check after 30 minutes if the mixture is separated. You need to check after every 30 minutes while cooking for 3 to 4 hours. Let this mixture cool and then add in a spray bottle.

Recipe 02: Coconut Soap

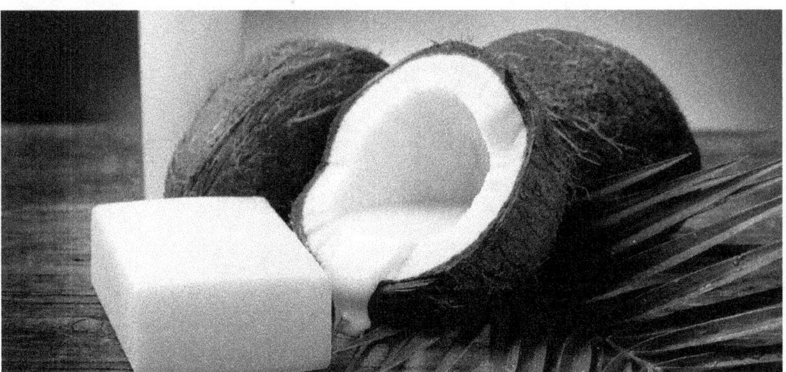

- Olive oil (40 percent)
- Lard (20 percent)
- Avocado oil (10 Percent)
- Castor oil (5 Percent)
- Coconut oil (25 Percent)
- Super-fast at 5 or better to have 6 percent

For 500g oils, the ingredients will be:
- 5 grams cocoa absolute
- 2 teaspoons Milk powder (whole milk)
- 2 teaspoons vanilla flecks
- 2 teaspoons coffee grains (instant)

- 1 tablespoon cocoa powder
- 2 teaspoons brownish clay (the rhassoul will be better)
- 2 teaspoons Reddish clay (the French red is better)
- 10 grams vanilla essential oil (10 folds)

Directions:

Follow the standard procedures of the soap manufacturing given in the first recipe. After becoming at the trace, you need to pour powders, clays, and essential oil. Pour the mixture into the mold and let it set for 24 hours. The expected age of the soap is almost 3 weeks, so enjoy.

Recipe 03: Butter and Sunflower Soap

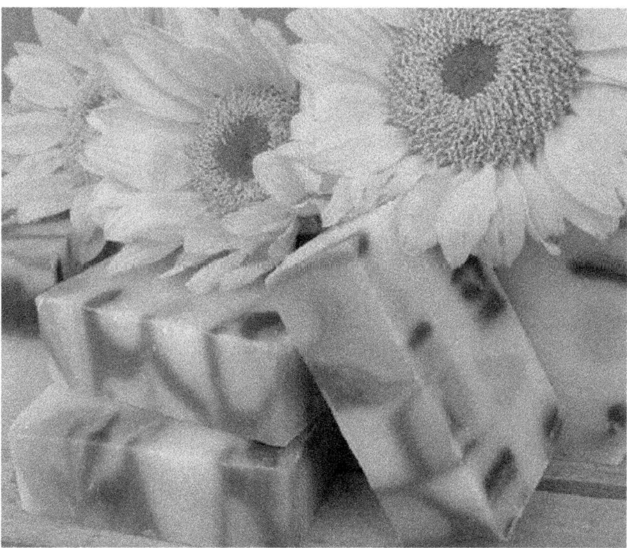

- 15-ounce sunflower oil
- 30-ounce coconut oil
- 5-ounce shea butter
- 18-ounce cucumber juice
- 27-ounce olive oil
- 21-ounce palm oil

- 19-ounce water
- 14.1-ounce lye (NaOH)
- Essential Oil

Directions:

Take cucumber juice and put it in a small pitcher. You can add colors and essential oils in the oils and lye during the cooling procedure. Follow the standard soap making procedures given in the first recipe.

Pour this mixture into the mold, insulate to let it set for 24 to 48 hours. After this particular time, you can unmold the soap and cut it. Keep it in the cookie rack and it is good to use for almost 4 weeks.

Recipe 04: Brass Cleanser

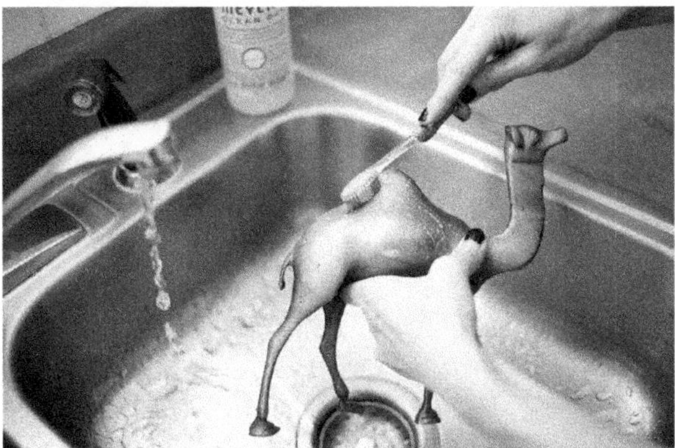

- Lemon juice or white vinegar
- Table salt

Procedure:

Damp one sponge with lemon juice or vinegar and sprinkle salt. Rub the surface and wash with water. Dry immediately with soft cloth.

Recipe 05: Marble Cleaner

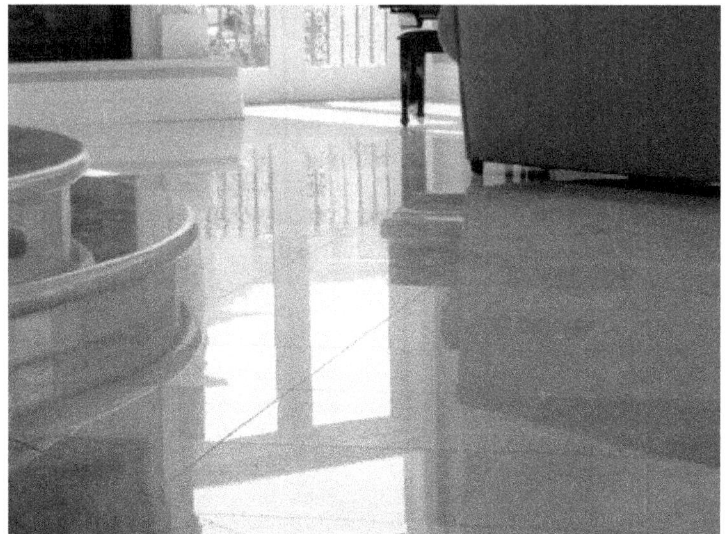

- Dishwashing liquid (mild): 2 drops
- Warm water: 2 cups

Procedure:

Mix water and detergent and use a sponge to clean marble. Wash with clean water and remove the residue of soap. You can buff with the help of one soft cloth to avoid water stains. You shouldn't let it air-dry. The lemon, vinegar, and acidic cleaner can eat your granite or marble.

Recipe 06: Cleaner and Toilets Deodorizers

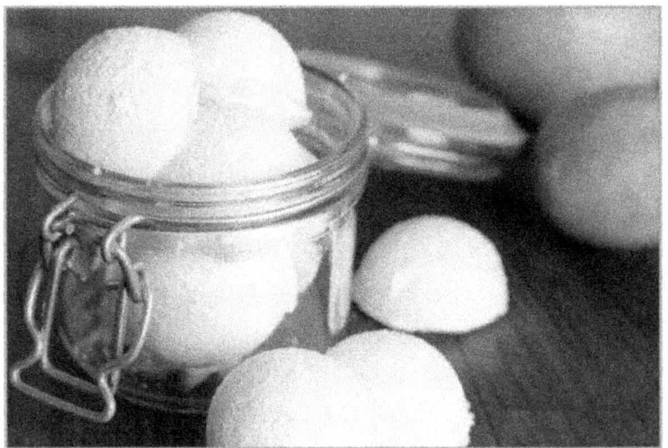

Pour only ½ cup baking soda and almost 10 drops of tea tree oil in your toilet. Add almost ¼ cup vinegar to this bowl and scrub away this mixture once it fizzes. For regular cleaning, you can fill a small spray bottle with 1 cup vinegar along with a few drops of essential oil and spray on the toilet seats. Leave it for a few minutes and wipe the surface to clean it.

If you want to clean shower and tub, you can use vinegar spray. Use this same mixture to spray shower and tub and leave for almost 30 minutes. Wash this surface with warm water and wipe with soft cloth. You can use baking soda with a bit of castile soap liquid for stubborn stains.

Recipe 07: Avocado Conditioner

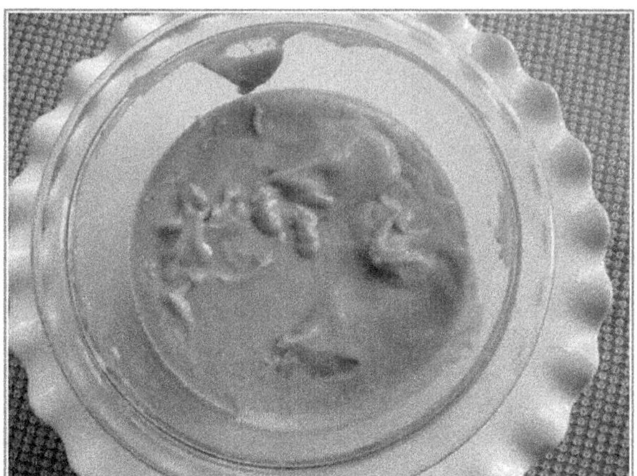

You will need Banana, Avocado, Eggs, Honey and Olive Oil (Extra Virgin).

Method: Peel and cut avocado and smash it to make a paste. If you have long hair then take full avocado and for short hair, the half avocado is enough. Take a banana and mix it well with the avocado paste. Add 2 tablespoons of olive oil and an egg to the mixture. Blend the mixture to make it soft.

Apply this mixture on the dry hair and start from the top section of your hair and apply the tips. It should not be applied on the scalp. Leave the mixture for almost 10 minutes on your scalp and then rinse with water. It will make your hair soft and shiny.

Recipe 08: Yogurt

If you have damaged hair, then use this recipe because the yogurt is an excellent conditioner for your locks. Egg white and Yogurt both are good for your damaged hair.

Thoroughly beat egg white only to make it smooth and then add six tablespoons of yogurt in the mixture. Blend the mixture well to make it smooth like a paste. Apply the blend to your hair and cover them with a shower cap for almost 15 to 30 minutes. Use a mild shampoo to wash your locks.

Recipe 09: Jojoba Oil

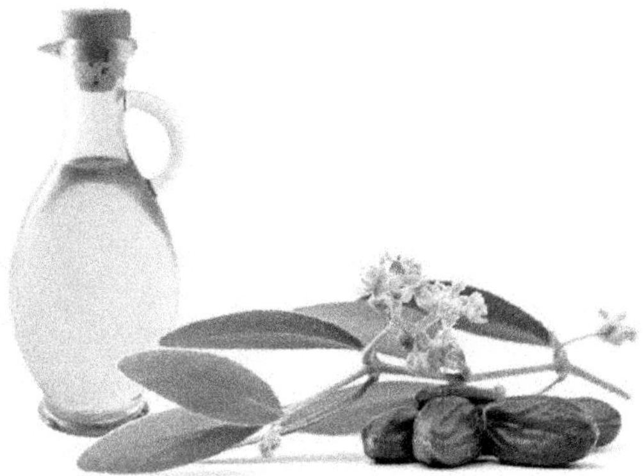

Ingredients: 2 teaspoons jojoba oil and 1 tablespoon organic soybean oil or sunflower oil

Mix the ingredients and keep them on a low heat to warm the oil. Test the temperature and massage this oil into locks. Take a hot towel and gently wrap your hair, but it is better to use a shower cap for 15 minutes. Use a mild shampoo and wash your locks after 15 minutes. It is an ideal recipe for those who want longer locks.

Recipe 10: Dandruff Treatment

The Fresh Ginger Roots, 1 teaspoon Sesame Oil and 1 teaspoon lemon juice are good ingredients for dandruff.

Extract the juice of ginger roots with the help of the press and mix all the ingredients to apply on the scalp. Leave for a few minutes to let it dry before using a mild shampoo. You need to repeat this recipe twice or thrice a week to get better results.

Recipe 11: Conditioner

You can take 1 small jar of mayonnaise and ½ avocado to condition your hair.
Peel and cut the avocado to mix it with mayonnaise in a small bowl with your hand. Mix it well to get a consistent green color and apply on the hair from top to end.

Cover your hair with a plastic wrap or a shower cap to seal the heat inside. Leave it for 20 minutes for deep conditioning. You can also use a hair dryer on low setting to give some heat to the wrap. 20 minutes, wash your hair with a mild shampoo.

Recipe 12: Homemade Conditioner

You can take ¼ cup distilled water, ¼ cup liquid Castile soap (scented or unscented), ½ teaspoon jojoba, grapeseed or other vegetable oil and Cap bottles or foaming bottles to make shampoo.

Prepare a mixture of all the ingredients and then store in a bottle. Shake well before use. The mixture is thin as compared to the commercial shampoos, so you can tilt the bottle on your head. Wake Up Your Scalp with Tea Tree Shampoo

Recipe 13: ALOE VERA

You can take the gel out of the aloe vera lead and use it on your hair. Simply rub it on your scalp then let it be for 30 minutes before you rinse it. If doing this once every week will let you have healthier and fuller hair. You can also eat flax seeds or hemp oil because they give your body essential fatty acids that are good for your hair growth.

Recipe 14: AVOCADO

Take half of a ripe avocado and mash it up. Then blend it in two tablespoons of olive oil and mix the combination. Apply the mixture to your hair and scalp and let it stay for 20 minutes. Then rinse and wash it out, and use a conditioner.

Recipe 15: CASTOR OIL

For re-growing hair, you can also use castor oil. It is extremely effective. Just add a few drops to your hair and massage your hair and scalp with it. Cover your head with a hair cap or towel and leave it there for around two hours. Wash it off with a shampoo and conditioner and notice immediate results.

Recipe 16: COCONUT OIL

Coconut oil is quite famous for healthy and thick hair, and rightfully so. A massage with coconut oil on your scalp will give you thicker locks in no time. Leave it on your hair for 30 minutes and cover your hair with a warm and moist towel. Repeat this process weekly and you will soon observe miraculous changes.

Recipe 17: FLAXSEEDS

Flaxseeds contain essential fatty acids such as omega-3 and omega-6 that are great for healthy hair growth. You can either eat them or soak a few tablespoons of seeds in water for 5 days and then apply the water solution on your head. Leave it on for ten minutes and then rinse it off.

Recipe 18: OLIVE OIL

You can also use olive oil to make your hair thicker. Apply it on your hair and scalp at night with a good massage and then go to sleep with a hair cap. Take a shower and wash your hair in the morning.

Recipe 19: PROTEIN

Proteins are great for your hair. Take enough in your diet to make sure your hair gets enough. You can also do a protein treatment by beating an egg, combined with yogurt and applying the mix on your hair.

Whisk an egg and add four tablespoons of grapes seed oil along with a few drops of lavender oil. Apply it on your scalp and hair and let it be for half an hour. Then rinse it out and wash thoroughly with shampoo.

Load up on foods rich in vitamin E such as red bell peppers, greens, broccoli, and spinach. Vitamin E promotes hair growth, makes it thicker and even prevents hair loss.

Chapter 2 – DIY Cleaning Products for Kitchen

Make your own cleaning products for your kitchen to save money and improve your health. You can use vinegar, baking soda, and water. These are simple and cheap ingredients without any chemical. You need bowl, sponge, spray bottle, scrub brush and measuring spoon to prepare kitchen cleaners:

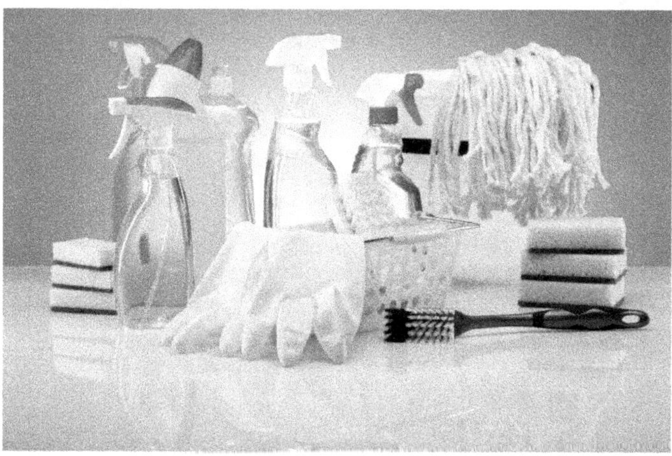

Essential Ingredients for Kitchen:
- Baking Soda
- Lemon
- Water
- Essential Oil
- Vinegar
- Dish Soap

Recipe 20: Freshener for Garbage Disposal

Take the pulp of one lemon (you can use already squeezed a lemon) and add it in your garbage disposal along with strips of lemon peel. Run water and now turn your disposal on.

Recipe 21: Dishwasher Detergent

- Washing soda: ¾ cup
- Lemi shine: ¾ cup
- Baking soda: ¼ cup
- Sea salt or Kosher: ¼ cup
-

Procedure:

Mix all ingredients in a bottle or mason jar and use 2 tablespoons in each load. You can add vinegar to rinse compartment.

Recipe 22: Microwave Cleaner

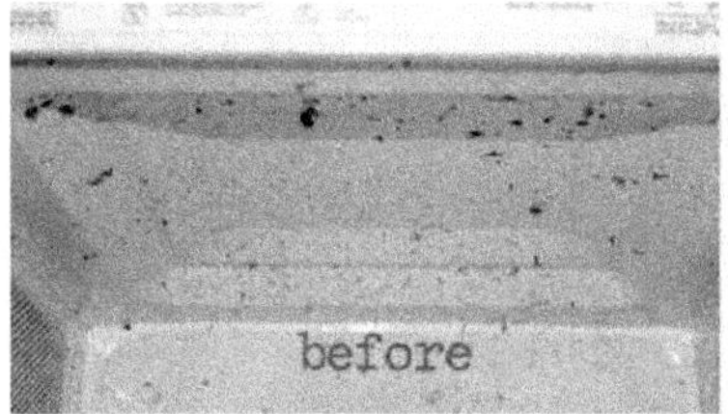

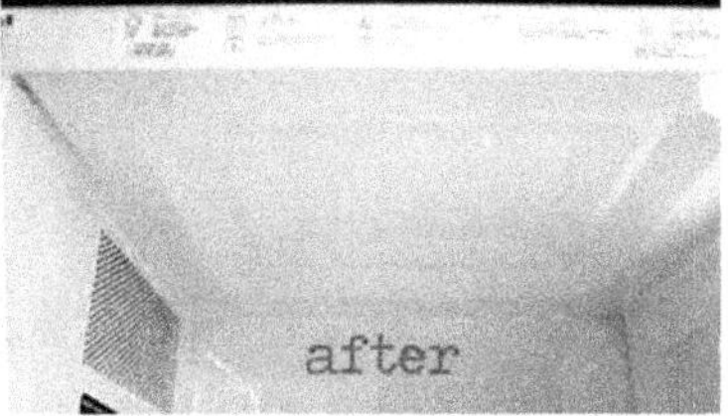

- Lemon: 1
- Microwave-safe bowl
- Cleaning rug and clean and dry dishtowel

Procedure:

Take a bowl and pour ½ cup water into this bowl. You can squeeze lemon juice in water and drop both lemon halves in this bowl. Put this bowl in microwave and microwave on high power for almost 3 minutes to let the liquid boil.

Don't open the door of the microwave for almost five minutes to let the steam loosen gunk of food.

Open the door and carefully take out the bowl with lemons. If you can turn the microwave, lift it and wipe to clean. Wipe the inside walls, sides and ceiling of your microwave and sweet crumbs in your hand. Carefully clean the door as well.

If you find any stubborn sport, you can dip the corner of your dishtowel in this lemon water and scrub the spot.

Recipe 23: Grease Cleaner

Ammonia mixed with water to make one container: ½ cups

Procedure:

Dip one sponge in solution and wipe the greased surface and use clear water to rinse this area.

Recipe 24: Use Coffee to Get Rid of Roaches

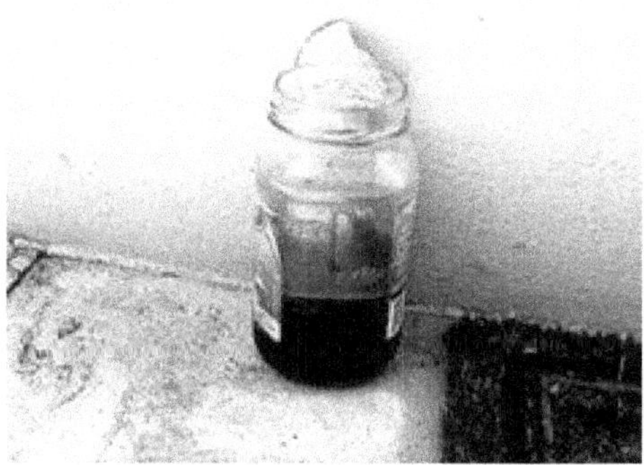

You can kill roaches with the help of coffee because perk and the smell of coffee are enough to kill roaches. You can mix coffee grinds in any organic edible and serve it to the roaches. It is really simple to do:

- You may fill the glass jar about halfway with water and place the coffee grinds in the small cups.

- Put a small cup in the one large glass jar and make 2 to 3 similar small cups in each jar.

- You can keep these jars near the nesting of roaches and on the places, where you frequently see the roaches.

- The odor of coffee will attract roaches and they may try to enter into the glass jar. Once the roaches fell into the jar of water, they will not be able to escape.

- Check the jar on a regular basis and toss them, once you have enough roaches in your jar.

- Replace the water and coffee to make a trap again for more roaches. You can continue this process to collect more roaches in the jar.

Recipe 25: Borax and Sugar Mixture

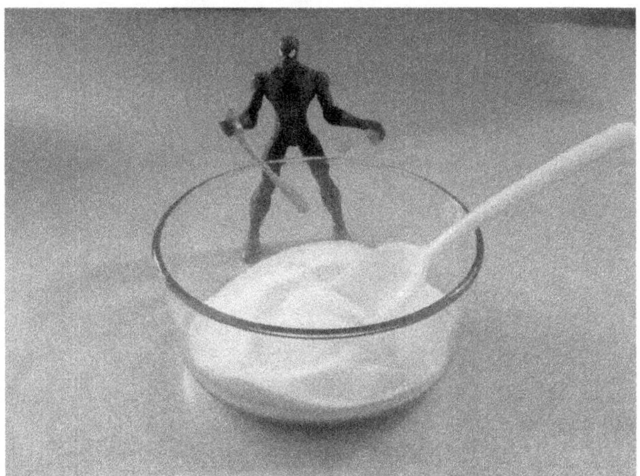

Roaches are usually attracted by organic things; therefore, you can use a mixture of borax and sugar to trap roaches. The borax is typically used in a commercial exterminator to kill roaches. The borax is harmful to the digestive system of cockroaches and dries out their exoskeleton. Get equal parts of sugar and borax to make this solution:

- Mix equal quantity of borax and sugar to serve roaches. Keep this mixture near the homes of roaches and apply this mixture on the homes of roaches.
- You can put this mixture into breaks, under cabinets, baseboards, and sink.
- You may see the dead roaches in a few hours after placing this mixture.

Borax powder is a toxic chemical; therefore, you should be careful while using this powder. Keep it away from your pets and kids. Sprinkle mixture carefully to keep it away from your pets and kids. Make sure to use gloves before making this mixture and wash your hands almost 2 to 3 times after completing your work.

Recipe 26: Cucumber Trap for Roaches

This remedy is really effective to remove roaches from your house. You can find a cucumber in your fridge and you can keep cucumber peels in an aluminum can to produce stink.

Aluminum can and cucumber may react to produce a particular stink and roaches will die off with this stink. For this trick, you will need fresh peels of cucumber and aluminum can:

- Take the aluminum can and place cucumber peels in it.
- Now, you can keep it near a place where you noticed numerous cockroaches.
- Wait for these pests to die away with its stink.

Recipe 27: Baking Soda and Sugar

You can make noxious bait with the help of baking soda and sugar to kill roaches. Baking soda is safer than borax; therefore, you can use it in a house with pets and children.

This bait is useful for your home because the sugar will attract the roaches and the baking soda will destroy their digestive system. Baking soda can create a great amount of gas into roaches and they will die:

- Take equal quantities of sugar and baking soda and prepare a mixture.
- Now, sprinkle this mixture in infested areas with roaches.
- Roaches will eat this mixture and die.

Recipe 28: Bay Leaf for Roaches

To push roaches away from your house, you can keep bay leaves in your house. It is a special herb and you can keep these herbs in your house.

The strong smell of bay leaves will keep the roaches away and they may not be able to enter in your house. This method is good for those people who want to get rid of cockroaches without killing them. You need a bunch of bay leaf and crush them with some tool:

- Take a bunch of bay leaves and let them dry. Crush these leaves and make a powder with the help of a tool.
- Sprinkle this powder near the nesting of roaches and they will leave their nests soon.

Recipe 29: Ammonia Water to Remove Roaches

Ammonia works very well to repel roaches because its sharp smell will keep roaches away from you. Prepare a propensity and clean the hard surfaces with the solution of water and ammonia. You need 1 bucket of water and 2 cups ammonia to prepare a mixture.

Wash your hard floor of bathroom and kitchen with this mixture and roaches will leave your house. It will be good to try it once in two weeks to keep your house free from roaches.

Recipe 30: Boric Acid for Roaches

This chemical is used by professionals to kill roaches because it is really effective. You can put boric acid on the top of bathroom and kitchen cabinets. You shouldn't keep them in cabinets because it is toxic.

Roaches are found in high places and you can keep boric acid on the top surface of your cabinets to keep them away. Roaches may take boric acid to home and kill their own species. You should keep this acid away from kids and pets and wash your hands properly after its use

Chapter 3 – All-purpose Cleaning Products

There are a few recipes that are easy to follow and the ingredients are already available in your kitchen. If some ingredients are missing, you can buy them from grocery stores:

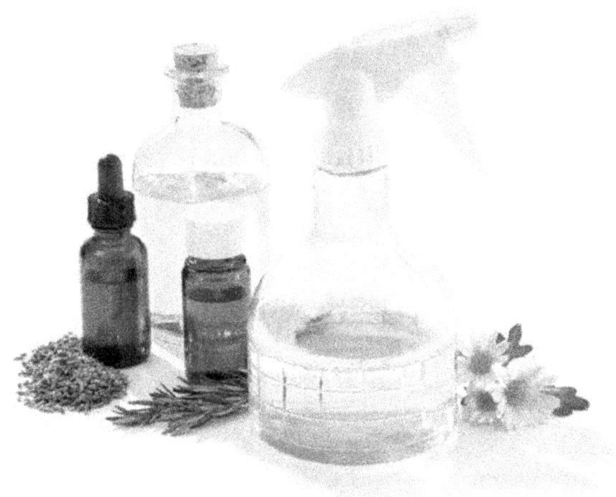

Recipe 31: All-purpose Cleaner
- Baking soda: ¼ cup
- Vinegar: ½ cup
- Water: ½ gallon

Procedure:

Mix all these ingredients together and pour into a spray bottle. This cleaner is efficient to clean glass.

Recipe 32: vinyl and linoleum
- Vinegar: 1 cup
- Baby oil: 3 drops

- Warm water: 1 gallon

Procedure:

Prepare a mixture with these ingredients and use it to clear linoleum and vinyl.

Recipe 33: Dusting Spray

- Olive oil: ¼ cup
- Lemon juice: 2 tablespoons

Procedure:

Combine all these ingredients in a spray bottle and shake well before use. Spray on one cloth and wipe down the surface. There is no need to spray on the furniture.

Recipe 34: Dusting Spray 02

- Castile soap: 1 tablespoon
- Lemon EO (essential oil): 15 drops
- Water: 2 cups

Procedure:

Pour all these ingredients in a spray bottle and shake them well to combine these ingredients. Spray this mixture on the surface and clean with one cloth.

Recipe 35: Furniture Polish

- Lemon: 1/8 cup
- Olive oil: ¼ cup
- White vinegar: 1 teaspoon

Directions:

Mix all these ingredients and mix them well to make a smooth solution. You can rub this polish on wood with a soft cloth that you may use for dusting. Rub the polish in wood to avoid oily surface.

Recipe 36: Wood Polish

- Water: ¾ cup
- Olive oil: 1 tablespoon
- White vinegar or vodka: 2 tablespoons

- White vinegar: 2 tablespoons
- Liquid glycerin: 1 tablespoon
- Orange, lemon or clove essential oil: 30 to 40 drops
- Xanthan gum: ¼ teaspoon
- Emulsifying wax (melted): ½ teaspoon

Directions:

Put water, essential oils, vodka, olive oil, glycerin and vinegar in one blender and blend these ingredients on high speed. While the motor is running, you can add emulsifying wax and xanthan gum. Process this mixture for almost 15 seconds to make it slightly thick. Pour in one spritz bottle and use once in a week. This can be kept for almost three months.

Recipe 37: Simple Dusting Spray

- Olive oil: ¾ cup
- Distilled vinegar (white): ¼ cup
- Essential oil (lemon, orange or clove): 30 to 40 drops

Procedure:

Put all ingredients in a spray bottle and shake forcefully. Spray on furniture and use a clean and dry cloth to buff this solution.

Recipe 38: Carpet Freshener

- Baking soda: 1 cup
- Essential oil (eucalyptus, lemon, and sweet orange): 10 to 20 drops
- Borax: ½ cup

Procedure:

Put all ingredients in a mason jar and shake well. Scoop this mixture into a cheese container or other container and shake well. Sprinkle this mixture on the carpet and wait for 15 minutes. Vacuum your carpet to enjoy the natural smell of disinfected carpet.

Recipe 39: Carpet Cleaner

- White Vinegar

- Lemon EO (essential oil): Optional
- Baking Soda
- Rags or old towels

Procedure:

If you want to use lemon EO, you have to blend it with baking soda and sprinkle this mixture on the spot. Let it sit for almost one hour or a whole night. If doesn't want to use essential oil, sprinkle plain soda on the stain. You have to mix 1:1 ratio of water and vinegar in one spray bottle. Spray this liquid mixture on baking soda and let the stain fizz. Put rag or towel on wet spot and press to completely absorb the moisture. If the stain is severe, you need to apply this mixture more than one time.

Recipe 40: Air Freshener

- Lavender EO (essential oil): ¾ teaspoon
- Sweet Orange EO: 1 teaspoon
- Lemon EO: ½ teaspoon

Procedure:

Add these essential oils in a spray bottle and pour water in this bottle. Mix them well to make a smooth blend. You should shake before every use and spray in the room.

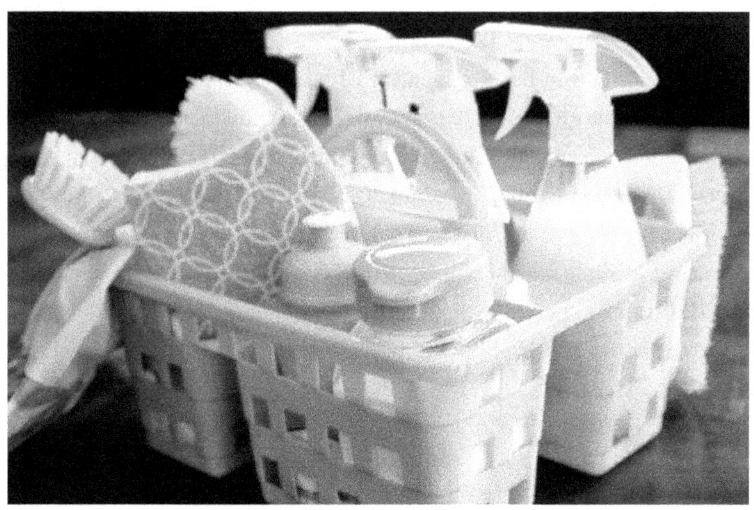

Recipe 41: Laundry Detergent

- Homemade Bar Soap (grated): 1 bar
- Washing soda: 1 cup
- Borax or washing soda: 1 cup
- Lemon EO (essential oil): 20 drops
- Oxygen booster: 1 cup

Procedure:

Use a food processor or hand grater to grate this soap. Grate soap into fine particles so that it can dissolve easily.

Carefully mix borax and washing soda together, but make sure to wear gloves or use a spoon to avoid any allergy problems on your skin. Mix essential oil and store this mixture in an air-tight jar. You can use almost 1 to 2 tablespoons in each load and add one tablespoon oxygen booster in white loads.

Recipe 42: Laundry Detergent Without Borax

- Washing soda: 1 cup

- Finely grated unscented glycerin soap: 1 bar
- Baking soda: ½ cup
- Citric acid: ½ cup
- Coarse salt: ¼ cup

Procedure:

Finely grate your bar of glycerin soap and add salt, citric acid, baking soda and washing soda in grated soap. Mix these ingredients and put one desiccant in a mason jar to avoid clumping. Store this mason jar in an airtight container. You can add 1 to 2 tablespoons determine to the machine to clean clothes.

Recipe 43: Fabric Softener

To make your clothes soft and nice, you can add 20 to 30 drops of any essential oil of your choice in one-gallon white vinegar. Mix them well and add 1/3 cup of this mixture in every laundry load. Shake this mixture well before sue.

Recipe 44: Laundry Scenter

If you want to get scented and clean laundry, you can use any one of dried herbs, such as lemon verbena, peppermint, and lavender. Add your favorite herb in a sachet and toss it in your dryer with clothes. You will get the non-toxic scent.

Recipe 45: Bleach

You can add some lemon juice in each load to clean all stains without chemicals. You can also use hydrogen peroxide, washing soda or borax. For general stains, you can use white vinegar or nontoxic soap.

Recipe 46: Laundry Soup

- Washing soda
- Borax
- Bar soap

Procedure:

Grate one bar soap and prepare a mixture in your food processor to ground it. You can use soap of your choice, such as coconut oil soap. You can also use Castile bar soap that is available in different scents, such as peppermint, lavender, almond, tea tree, etc.

Take a large bowl and add 2 parts borax, 2 parts soda (washing soda) and grated soap (1 part). Add a few teaspoons baking soda. Mix them well and store in a closed mason jar or container. Use 1/8 – ¼ cup in each load of your laundry.

Recipe 47: Laundry Soap Procedure

If you want to make soap at home, it is important to know the standard soap making procedures:

- It is important to weigh all your ingredients and it will be good to use the tare function on the digital scale to get the weight of the containers.
- Lye solution will be prepared by putting weighted water in a pot or a bowl of stainless steel. Carefully include lye in the water and stir it continuously. As a reaction, the heating up of the water will be started. Make sure to avoid boiling of water and don't swallow the fumes. Keep it one side to let it cool.
- During the cooling process of the lye, you can take a stainless steel pan and put in the sufficient quantity of oils to the pan. Let the oils melt on a slow heat.
- Measure the temperatures of oils and the lye mixture. The ideal temperature may be 100 to 125 F ranges and slowly mix the lye solution into the oils.
- Mix them gently and then add color after getting a smooth texture. You can blend this mixture in the blender for almost 20 seconds.
- At a particular point, your blend will reach trace. The trace is a situation in which the surface of the solution may show waves on the surface. It will look like thick custard.
- You may add oils, dyes, fragrances and additives at the time of its completion, before adding into molds.

- Pour this mixture into the molds and leave for almost 24 hours to let the molds sit. Cover them with a blanket or lid for 24 hours. After 24 hours, you need to remove the lid and let the air circulates in the mold for a few hours.

- You will get a beautiful hard block of the organic soap and now you can remove them from the mold. It will be a bit soft, but leaves in one day to let it sit. You can cut the soap in the small bars and don't let them stick with one another. Keep turning the bars regularly and you will be able to try the soap after 2 weeks or more.

Recipe 48: Liquid Laundry Soap

Take a soap bar and process it in a food processor or use a cheese grater. Put soap in your pan with two quarts water on low heat and stir constantly to completely dissolve soap.

Put almost 4.5 gallons of hot tap water in a 5-gallon bucket and mix two cups of washing soda and two cups borax in this water. Mix them well and pour soap mixture in this 5-gallon bucket. Mix them well and cover for one night. Shake well until smooth and pour into containers. You can use ½ - 1 cup in each load.

Recipe 49: Stovetop Cleaner

Take a bowl and add 1/3 cup baking soda and mix it with warm water. You should make a nice paste and put this paste on your brush or sponge. Scrub the surface with this mixture.

Recipe 50: Peppermint Shampoo

You need to take ¼ cup distilled water, ¼ cup liquid Castile soap, 2 teaspoon jojoba oil, 1/8 teaspoon peppermint essential oil, 1/8 teaspoon tea tree essential oil and Flip cap or foaming bottles.

Mix all the ingredients well and then add ¼ cup distilled water. Secure the shampoo in a bottle and use it just like a shampoo. Wash your hair well after applying it.

Conclusion

Herbs like rosemary, burdock, nettle, catnip, sage and horsetail help you grow hair faster. If you want your hair to grow out quickly, then rosemary, in particular, is an excellent choice. Besides faster hair growth, it also adds luster to your locks.

Moreover, green tea has polyphenols and anti-inflammatory properties that are linked to hair growth and they improve circulation as well.

Make yourself an herbal infusion by adding any of these herbs in hot water for 10 to 20 minutes and then use it as a final rinse after the process of shampoo and conditioning. You can also start drinking herbal tea regularly. You can use all these recipes because these are free from toxins and good for your family members.

www.ingramcontent.com/pod-product-compliance
Lightning Source LLC
Chambersburg PA
CBHW061930270726
48660CB00003BA/1117